Structured Interview for DSM-IV Personality

SIDP-IV

Bruce Pfohl, M.D.

Nancee Blum, M.S.W.

Mark Zimmerman, M.D.

Name _____ # _____ Date ___/___/___

Structured Interview for DSM-IV Personality

SIDP-IV

Department of Psychiatry
The University of Iowa

Bruce Pfohl, M.D.

Nancee Blum, M.S.W.

Mark Zimmerman, M.D.

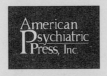

American Psychiatric Press, Inc.

Washington, DC
London, England

Books published by the American Psychiatric Press, Inc., represent the views and opinions of the individual authors and do not necessarily represent the policies and opinions of the Press or the American Psychiatric Association.

Copyright © 1997 Bruce Pfohl, Nancee Blum, and Mark Zimmerman
ALL RIGHTS RESERVED. No part of this instrument may be reproduced or transmitted in any form or by any means, electronic or mechanical, including photocopying, or by any information storage or retrieval system, without permission in writing from the publisher.

Manufactured in the United States of America on acid-free paper
11 10 09 08   4 3 2

American Psychiatric Press, Inc.
1000 Wilson Blvd.
Arlington, VA 22209
www.appi.org

ISBN 0-88048-937-5

INTRODUCTION AND BACKGROUND

Since its introduction in 1983, versions of the SIDP have been used in numerous studies at many different centers and translated into several different languages. We are aware of more than 60 publications using the SIDP and SIDP-R. We are therefore pleased to present this revision keyed to DSM-IV. As before, we have endeavored to formulate nonpejorative questions that address what the personality traits look like from the perspective of the individual experiencing them. Another aim has been to inquire about a range of behaviors that illustrate a trait rather than merely asking the subject's opinion about whether the trait is present. Where appropriate, the interviewer is cued to look beyond the content of the subject's responses and consider the overall pattern of interaction during the interview.

As with previous versions, the SIDP-IV is organized into topical sections rather than by disorder. This allows for a more natural conversational flow and increases the likelihood that useful information from related questions may be taken into account when rating related criteria within that section. Unlike previous versions, the rater is given the opportunity to rate or at least refer to the specific DSM-IV criterion associated with each set of questions. This change resulted from our observations that experienced SIDP raters obtained the best results by keeping the specific criterion in mind as associated questions were asked.

Once an interviewer is familiar with the instrument, the subject interview can be completed in 60–90 minutes; an additional 20 minutes is usually required if an informant is interviewed and 20–30 minutes to rate the sections and fill in the scoresheet. While the interview time varies considerably due to patient/subject variables, the skill and experience of the interviewer also play a major role.

There are several options for customizing and shortening the SIDP-IV interview. First, the optional diagnoses (Self-Defeating Personality Disorder, Depressive Personality Disorder, and Negativistic Personality Disorder) can easily be omitted, since the questions for these disorders are grouped at the end of each topical section. Second, many studies already screen for antisocial personality using some other assessment tool e.g., the DIS). If this is the case, the questions for

antisocial personality disorder can be omitted from Section J (Social Conformity). Finally, for clinicians who simply wish to systematically evaluate for presence or absence of one or more specific personality disorders, a modular version of the SIDP-IV is available in which the criteria are listed by disorder rather than by topic. Only those personality disorders of specific interest need be assessed.

INTERVIEWING INSTRUCTIONS

The SIDP-IV is intended to follow a general psychiatric interview and/or chart review in which episodic psychiatric disorders have been assessed. This helps the interviewer more easily distinguish lifelong behavior reported by the patient from temporary states due to an episodic psychiatric disorder. Although the patient is repeatedly reminded to answer according to *what you are like when you are your usual self,* it may be necessary to clarify this issue with additional questions. For example, overdependency during discrete episodes of depression does not count. On the other hand, if the patient has had angry verbal outbursts several times a month for many years that are not explained by discrete episodes of psychiatric disorder, this would count as *lack of control of anger,* even if the patient considered such behavior not to be part of his/her usual self.

To ensure accurate recall of information, the rater should write in the patient's response next to each question on the interview form. In some cases this can be a simple *yes* or *no,* but a short phrase or example of the behavior is always preferable. If the answer to a given question was already obtained as part of a response to a previous question, then the answer can be written beside that question without taking time to ask it. Questions should not be skipped because the interviewer suspects the answer will be unrevealing. *ALL QUESTIONS MUST HAVE SOME RESPONSE WRITTEN IN THE MARGIN.* Since the SIDP-IV is a semistructured interview, it may sometimes be necessary to probe further with questions that go beyond those provided in the interview.

For each criterion, a rating of 0, 1, 2, or 3 is possible. At a minimum, the interviewer should silently read over the criterion before moving on to the next set of questions in order to verify that sufficient information has been elicited to make a rating. Some experienced raters prefer to pencil in a tentative rating during the subject interview, but a final rating should always be postponed until all sources of information have been reviewed.

If an individual's personality has changed dramatically in recent years, the personality which has predominated for the *greatest amount of time in the last 5 years* should be considered typical.

INTERVIEWING AN INFORMANT

Use of an informant is optional. A consent form for contacting a third party is provided at the end of the interview. Family members and very close friends are the most desirable informants. The same interview should be used for the informant, but a different-color ink should be used to record responses. Questions will need to be rephrased, changing second person pronouns to third person. Suitable follow-up questions may need to be composed or adapted from existing probes to clarify the informant's answer.

The interviewer should, at a minimum, ask those questions that are preceded by an asterisk (*). If the answers to those questions reveal new information that was not obtained from the patient, then additional questions from that section should be asked.

Confidentiality requires that the patient's responses not be revealed to the informant and vice versa. Previous research suggests that the addition of informant information generally increases the frequency of personality diagnoses but that predictive validity is neither increased nor decreased.

RATING INSTRUCTIONS

Final rating should be delayed until all sources of information have been reviewed. Depending on your protocol, this could include patient and informant interviews, review of hospital records, and other clinical evaluations.

Start at the beginning of the interview and work through each criterion in the order it was asked during the interview, coding each criterion as 0, 1, 2, or 3 by circling the appropriate number. Additional rating guidelines in bold should be followed where indicated.

There are several complications that may arise in determining whether a given criterion is part of an

enduring pattern that is stable and of long duration, with onset *traced back at least to adolescence or early adulthood*. If the individual is several decades past early adulthood, it may be difficult to get accurate retrospective information. Several studies show that even patients with severe borderline personality disorder may no longer meet criteria for this disorder when followed up a decade later. Episodic Axis I disorders may temporarily alter usual interpersonal functioning, yet it is not uncommon for personality disorders to be comorbid with major depression, substance abuse, etc.

To operationalize such decisions, the SIDP has always used the *5-year rule*. This means that the behavior, cognitions, and feelings that have predominated for most of the last 5 years are considered to be representative of the individual's long-term personality functioning. An individual's behavior during an episode of major depression would not be considered representative of his or her long-term personality functioning as long as that behavior has not been typical of their functioning for most of the last 5 years. On the other hand, a patient with a several-year history of symptoms typical of a personality disorder (e.g., borderline personality disorder) who has also been chronically depressed for most of the last 5 years would be scored as having the traits for the personality diagnosis. A patient with a history of symptoms of a personality disorder that has remitted with time (or with therapy) would no longer be rated as meeting the criteria for that disorder when the symptoms have been absent for most of the past 5 years. In our experience, the 5-year rule satisfactorily operationalizes a complex set of clinical decisions that would otherwise lead to considerable unreliability. Cases with overwhelming Axis I pathology (e.g., schizophrenia, severe bipolar disorder, organic brain disorders) would still be excluded from personality diagnosis by Criterion E of the General Diagnostic Criteria for Personality Disorder (GCPD) (see scoresheet).

After all the criteria have been rated, return to the beginning of the interview and transfer each rating to the scoresheet at the end of the manual. The scoresheet can be detached for easier coding. Even if a given criterion is not present, a 0 or 1 should be transferred to the scoresheet. The scoresheet is then reviewed to make sure all criteria have been scored.

The General Diagnostic Criteria for Personality Disorder (GCPD) are then rated based on all sources of information. Criterion D will generally be operationalized using the 5-year rule unless your specific study protocol specifies otherwise.

Finally, each personality disorder on the scoresheet should be reviewed to determine if sufficient criteria are present (i.e., scored 2 or 3) to meet the minimum number of criteria necessary. If this is the case, and if the GCPD criteria are met, a 1 is entered in the square brackets and the diagnosis is circled on the scoresheet; otherwise, a 0 is entered. The exclusion criteria for a personality diagnosis are incorporated into the GCPD assessment, except for the case of antisocial personality disorder where criteria B and C must also be met.

TRAINING FOR INTERVIEWERS

The SIDP-IV interview is technically a semistructured interview since the interviewer may need to probe with additional questions at times to clarify the patient's responses. The ability to clarify with additional questions and to discriminate between Axis I and Axis II disorders requires that the interviewer have some awareness of the criteria and typical course of the major Axis I diagnoses. The authors have obtained good results with interviewers whose minimum training consists of an undergraduate degree in the social sciences plus 6 months previous experience in interviewing psychiatric patients. A person with this level of experience generally takes about 1 month of training to become a competent interviewer.

Investigators are reminded that attributes such as reliability and validity are not attached to an interview directly but are unique to a specific set of interviewers and a specific target population. It is important that each new study incorporate some measure of reliability and validity. Inquiries about on-site training, reliability assessments, computer scoring aids, and training tapes should be addressed to Nancee Blum, MSW, or Bruce Pfohl, MD, Department of Psychiatry, University of Iowa College of Medicine, Iowa City, Iowa, 52242. Phone: 319-353-6180. FAX: 319-356-2587. Email: <bruce-pfohl@uiowa.edu> or <nancee-blum@uiowa.edu>. Relevant citations, foreign-language versions, and other SIDP-IV information are available on the Internet at http://ourworld.compuserve.com/homepages/Bruce_P/SIDP

INTRODUCTION TO SIDP-IV INTERVIEW

I would like to ask you some questions about the way you think and act in a variety of situations. I am most interested in what you are like when you are your usual self. If you are currently hospitalized or experiencing an illness, please try to remember what you are like when you are your usual self.

I am going to ask you all the questions in this booklet. With your permission, I would like to ask someone who knows you well some of the same questions that I ask you. This usually takes 15-20 minutes and can be done by telephone. Your answers and theirs will be totally confidential. Is there someone you would be willing to let me talk with?

■ **(IF SUBJECT AGREES, ASK HIM/HER TO SIGN CONSENT FORM ON PAGE 34)**

Scoring Guidelines:
0=not present or limited to rare isolated examples
*1=subthreshold — some evidence of the trait, but it is not sufficiently
pervasive or severe to consider the criterion present*
*2=present — criterion is clearly present for most of the last 5 years (i.e.,
present at least 50% of the time during the last 5 years)*
*3=strongly present — criterion is associated with subjective distress or
some impairment in social or occupational functioning or
intimate relationships*

A. INTERESTS AND ACTIVITIES

The first part of this interview asks about your interests and activities. Remember that I am interested in the way you are when you are your usual self.

---

1. **Takes pleasure in few, if any, activities**   4-SZOID   0   1   2   3

What kinds of things do you enjoy?
(IF ONLY 1 OR 2 ARE MENTIONED):
If [*list activities mentioned*] were not available, are
there other things you would enjoy doing?

---

2. **Almost always chooses solitary activities**   2-SZOID   0   1   2   3

* Some people prefer to spend time with other people, while
others prefer to work and do things alone. How would you
describe yourself?
(IF ALONE): Do you almost always choose to do things by
yourself?

---

3. **Is unusually reluctant to take personal risks or to engage in any new activities**   7-AVOID   0   1   2   3
because they may prove embarrassing

Do you usually avoid taking chances or trying new activities
because you're worried about embarrassing yourself?
(IF YES):   Examples?

**4. Has difficulty making everyday decisions without an excessive amount of advice   1-DEPEN   0 1 2 3
and reassurance from others**

Some people enjoy making decisions and other people prefer
to have someone they trust tell them what to do. Which do you
prefer?

*   Do you often turn to others for advice about everyday
decisions like what to have for lunch or what clothes to buy?

5.   Needs others to assume responsibility for most major areas of his or her life   2-DEPEN   0 1 2 3

*   Some people turn to others to make decisions about important
areas of their life. For example, they let someone else decide
whether they should take a job, who their friends should be,
etc. Does this sound like your life?
    (IF YES): What keeps you from making decisions on your
                own?

**6.   Has difficulty initiating projects or doing things on his or her own (because of a   4-DEPEN   0 1 2 3
lack of self-confidence in judgment or abilities rather than a lack of motivation or
energy)**

Do you usually need help from somebody else to get started on
a project or do things on your own?
    (IF YES): Why is that?
                (IF UNCLEAR): Is it because you don't feel
                            confident about your own
                            abilities?

**7.   Adopts a miserly spending style toward both self and others; money is viewed as   7-OBCMP   0 1 2 3
something to be hoarded for future catastrophes**

After you pay your bills, what kinds of things do you like to
spend money on?

Are you slow to spend money on yourself?

Are you slow to spend money on others?

*   Some people worry so much about something terrible
happening in the future, that they hold on to all their money.
Does this sound like you?
    (IF YES): Tell me about that.

▐ **(SKIP TO SECTION B IF OPTIONAL DIAGNOSES ARE NOT BEING ASSESSED)**

0=not present, 1=subthreshold, 2=present, 3=strongly preser

8. **Rejects opportunities for pleasure, or is reluctant to acknowledge enjoying himself or herself (despite having adequate social skills and the capacity for pleasure)**   5-SLFDF   0 1 2 3

When you have a chance to do something that's fun, is it hard to enjoy it?

Is it hard for you to admit that you've had a good time?
   (IF YES TO EITHER):
          Have you always been this way?
          What keeps you from enjoying things?

Do you usually turn down opportunities to have a good time?
   (IF YES): Why is this?

> **Scoring Guidelines:**
> 0=not present or limited to rare isolated examples
> 1=subthreshold — some evidence of the trait, but it is not sufficiently
>   pervasive or severe to consider the criterion present
> 2=present — criterion is clearly present for most of the last 5 years (i.e.,
>   present at least 50% of the time during the last 5 years)
> 3=strongly present — criterion is associated with subjective distress or
>   some impairment in social or occupational functioning or
>   intimate relationships

B. WORK STYLE

The questions in this section are concerned with your work style. This can include either a job outside the home or doing household chores.

---

1. **Is excessively devoted to work and productivity to the exclusion of leisure activities and friendships (not accounted for by obvious economic necessity)**   3-OBCMP   0 1 2 3

---

* Would you call yourself a workaholic?

Have others complained about how much time you spend working?
   (IF YES TO EITHER):
      Has your devotion to work left you with little time
      for family activities, friendships, or entertainment?

---

2. **Avoids occupational activities that involve significant interpersonal contact, because of fears of criticism, disapproval, or rejection**   1-AVOID   0 1 2 3

Do you enjoy a job that requires a lot of interaction with other people, or do you try to avoid that kind of work?
   (IF AVOIDS): Why is that?
      (IF UNCLEAR): Are you afraid that people
               will criticize or reject you?

Have you ever turned down a job or promotion because it involved more contact with people?
   (IF YES): Why is that?

---

3. **Is interpersonally exploitative, i.e., takes advantage of others to achieve his or her own ends**   6-NARCI   0 1 2 3

Are you pretty good at getting people to do what you want?
  (IF YES): How do you get them to do what you want?
           Do you ever pretend you like someone so they'll do
           something for you?

Have you ever taken advantage of someone because it was the
only way to get what you needed or deserved?
  (IF YES): Can you describe a situation?
           How often have you done something like this?

* Do you have a reputation for doing whatever it takes to get
what you want, even if it means stepping on other people?

---

4. **Shows perfectionism that interferes with task completion (e.g., is unable to complete a project because his or her own overly strict standards are not met)**   2-OBCMP   0 1 2 3

Would people describe you as a perfectionist?

Do you think you are a perfectionist?
  (IF YES TO EITHER):
        How often do your high standards keep you from
        getting projects completed on time?
        Examples?

---

5. **Is reluctant to delegate tasks or to work with others unless they submit to exactly his or her way of doing things**   6-OBCMP   0 1 2 3

---

* Do you end up doing a lot of jobs yourself because no one else
will do it exactly the way you want it done?

Do you often take over other people's responsibilities to make
sure things get done right?
  (IF YES): Examples?

---

6. **Is preoccupied with details, rules, lists, order, organization, or schedules to the extent that the major point of the activity is lost**   1-OBCMP   0 1 2 3

---

* When you're working on something, do you often spend so
much time on small details that you lose sight of the main
point?
  (IF YES): Examples?

Do you often spend so much time getting organized, that you
have trouble getting a task done?

Has anyone ever told you that you spend too much time
making lists and schedules of what you need to do?

Do you think you do?

■ (SKIP TO SECTION C IF OPTIONAL DIAGNOSES ARE NOT BEING ASSESSED)

---

7. Passively resists fulfilling routine social and occupational tasks   1-NEGTV   0 1 2 3

When some people get tired of doing their daily chores at work
or at home, they might try to get out of them by inventing
excuses, pretending to forget, or deliberately not working very
hard. Do you often do things like this?
  (IF YES): Have others complained about this?

**8. Fails to accomplish tasks crucial to his or her personal objectives despite
demonstrated ability to do so, e.g., helps fellow students write papers, but is
unable to write his/her own**   6-SLFDF   0 1 2 3

Some people are able to do things for others, but can't do the
same thing for themselves. For example, they'll do someone
else's work at their job, and not get their own work done. Is
this something you do?
  (IF YES): Examples?

Do you often set goals but then fail to reach them, even though
you have the ability to do it?
  (IF YES): Examples?
          What seems to get in the way?

---

9. Rejects or renders ineffective the attempts of others to help him or her   2-SLFDF   0 1 2 3

---

* Is it hard for you to accept help from others, even when you
know you need it?
  (IF YES): Even though it is hard, do you usually accept help?
          Can you describe some situations where you
          refused the help you needed?

When you let people help you, do you find yourself trying to
convince them that it won't work?
  (IF YES): Tell me about it.

0=not present, 1=subthreshold, 2=present, 3=strongly present

> **Scoring Guidelines:**
> *0=not present or limited to rare isolated examples*
> *1=subthreshold — some evidence of the trait, but it is not sufficiently*
> * pervasive or severe to consider the criterion present*
> *2=present — criterion is clearly present for most of the last 5 years (i.e.,*
> * present at least 50% of the time during the last 5 years)*
> *3=strongly present — criterion is associated with subjective distress or*
> * some impairment in social or occupational functioning or*
> * intimate relationships*

C. CLOSE RELATIONSHIPS

This part of the interview asks about your relationships with friends and family. Remember that I'm interested in the way you are when you are your usual self.

---

1. Neither desires nor enjoys close relationships, including being part of a family   1-SZOID 0 1 2 3

---

* Do you have close relationships with friends or family?
  (IF YES): What do you enjoy about these relationships?
  (IF NO): Do you wish you had some close relationships?

---

2. Lacks close friends or confidants other than first-degree relatives   5-SZOID 0 1 2 3
                                8-STYPL

Not counting your immediate family, do you have close friends you can confide in?

---

3. Shows restraint within intimate relationships because of the fear of being shamed or ridiculed   3-AVOID 0 1 2 3

In a close relationship, do you often keep your thoughts and feelings to yourself because you're afraid the other person might put you down?
  (IF YES): How much has this fear kept you from sharing your
         true feelings in close relationships?

---

4. Has difficulty expressing disagreement with others because of fear of loss of support or approval (NOTE: Do not include realistic fears of retribution)   3-DEPEN 0 1 2 3

How hard is it for you to disagree with someone?
  (IF HARD): What are you afraid might happen if you do?

* Do you often pretend to agree with others so they won't reject you or dislike you?

5. **A pattern of unstable and intense interpersonal relationships characterized by alternating between extremes of idealization and devaluation**   2-BORDL   0 1 2 3

Do your relationships with friends and lovers tend to be
intense and stormy with lots of ups and downs?
    (IF YES): Can you tell me about some of them?

* Do you switch from loving and admiring people at one time, to
hating them at another time?
    (IF YES): How often has this happened?

---

6. **Is unrealistically preoccupied with fears of being left to take care of himself or herself**   8-DEPEN   0 1 2 3

Do you worry about the people you depend on leaving you?
    (IF YES):   Are there times when you can't stop worrying
               about this?
               What has caused your concern?
               Are you worried that you won't be able to
               take care of yourself?

---

7. **Frantic efforts to avoid real or imagined abandonment. [NOTE: Do not include suicidal or self-mutilating behavior covered in Criterion 5]**   1-BORDL   0 1 2 3

* Have there been times when you've been very upset because
you thought someone might leave you?
    (IF YES): What have you done to keep them from leaving?
          (IF ONLY SUICIDAL/SELF-MUTILATING BEHAVIOR):
               What else have you done?

Do you spend a lot of time thinking of ways to keep people
from leaving you?

---

8. **Urgently seeks another relationship as a source of care and support when a close relationship ends**   7-DEPEN   0 1 2 3

What do you do when a close relationship ends?

Would you be desperate to get into another relationship right
away, even if it was not the best person for you?
    (IF YES): Why is that?

0=not present, 1=subthreshold, 2=present, 3=strongly present

9. **Has recurrent suspicions, without justification, regarding fidelity of spouse or sexual partner**   7-PARND   0 1 2 3

When you're in a relationship, do you often worry that your partner is unfaithful to you?
   (IF EVER):   Has that person done anything to make you suspicious?
                    Have you ever had proof that a partner was unfaithful?

10. **Has little, if any, interest in having sexual experiences with another person**   3-SZOID   0 1 2 3

In general, has your sex life been important to you, or could you have gotten along as well without it?
   (IF SAYS NOT IMPORTANT OR NOT CURRENTLY INVOLVED):
                    Would it bother you to live your entire life without sexual relationships?

■ **(SKIP TO SECTION D IF OPTIONAL DIAGNOSES ARE NOT BEING ASSESSED)**

11. **Chooses people and situations that lead to disappointment, failure, or mistreatment even when better options are clearly available**   1-SLFDF   0 1 2 3

Do you seem to get yourself into situations where you get treated badly?
   (IF YES): Examples?
                 Does it seem like this has been a pattern for you?
                 What makes it hard to avoid these situations?

* Does it seem like most of the people you choose to get involved with disappoint you or let you down?
   (IF YES): Examples?

Have you ever left one bad relationship only to end up with someone else who was just as bad?
   (IF YES): Has this happened more than once?

12. **Is uninterested in or rejects people who consistently treat him or her well, e.g., is unattracted to caring sexual partners**   7-SLFDF   0 1 2 3

Do you have trouble maintaining relationships with people who treat you better than you think you deserve?
   (IF YES): How often has this happened?

> **Scoring Guidelines:**
> *0=not present or limited to rare isolated examples*
> *1=subthreshold — some evidence of the trait, but it is not sufficiently pervasive or severe to consider the criterion present*
> *2=present — criterion is clearly present for most of the last 5 years (i.e., present at least 50% of the time during the last 5 years)*
> *3=strongly present — criterion is associated with subjective distress or some impairment in social or occupational functioning or intimate relationships*

D. SOCIAL RELATIONSHIPS

The next set of questions concerns the way you think and act in situations that involve other people.

---

1. Views self as socially inept, personally unappealing, or inferior to others   **6-AVOID**   0 1 2 3

How do you think you relate to people in social situations?

Even when you're at your best, do you usually feel like you're not as much fun to be around as other people?

---

2. Is uncomfortable in situations in which he or she is not the center of attention   **1-HISTR**   0 1 2 3

* Some people prefer to be the center of attention, while others are content to remain on the edge of things. Where would you put yourself?
   (IF CENTER):   How do you feel when you're not the center of attention?

---

3. Interaction with others is often characterized by inappropriate sexually seductive or provocative behavior   **2-HISTR**   0 1 2 3

* Do you have a reputation for being a flirt?
   (IF YES): Tell me about that.

Do people sometimes misinterpret your friendliness as a romantic or sexual invitation?
   (IF YES): How often does that happen?

■ **(RATING NOTE: ALSO CONSIDER BEHAVIOR DURING INTERVIEW)**

---

4.   Consistently uses physical appearance to draw attention to self   4-HISTR   0 1 2 3

Compared to other people your age, are you more interested
in having your appearance noticed?

*   How often do you use your appearance to get people's
attention?
   (IF OFTEN):   How do you do that?

Are you disappointed when people don't notice how you look?

▌ **(RATING NOTE: ALSO CONSIDER APPEARANCE DURING INTERVIEW)**

**5.   Believes that he or she is "special" and unique and can only be understood by,   3-NARCI   0 1 2 3
or should associate with, other special or high-status people (or institutions)**

Some people are so creative and unique that they have a hard
time finding people like themselves to share things with. Does
this sound like you?
   (IF YES):   What kind of person is able to understand you and
                be a good friend?

---

6.   Is inhibited in new interpersonal situations because of feelings of inadequacy   5-AVOID   0 1 2 3

Do you have a lot more trouble than most people carrying on a
conversation with someone you've just met?
   (IF YES):   What makes it hard?
                (IF UNCLEAR): Is it because you think you don't
                measure up?

Are you often very shy and quiet in new social situations?

**7.   Excessive social anxiety that does not diminish with familiarity and tends to be   9-STYPL   0 1 2 3
associated with paranoid fears rather than negative judgments about self**

---

*   Do you generally feel nervous or anxious around people?
   (IF YES):   How bad does it get?
                Do you get nervous around people because you
                worry about what they might be up to, or is it
                because you don't feel you're as good as other
                people?

                Are you less nervous after you get to know people
                better?

---

8.   Is unwilling to get involved with people unless certain of being liked   2-AVOID   0 1 2 3

How often do you avoid getting to know people because you're
worried they may not like you?
   (IF OFTEN):   Has this affected the number of friends you
                have?

9. **Is reluctant to confide in others because of unwarranted fear that the information will be used maliciously against him or her** 3-PARND 0 1 2 3

Do you believe there's often a price to pay if you share
something personal with others?
   (IF YES): Does this keep you from opening up to others?
                  What might happen if you did confide?

10. **Lacks empathy: is unwilling to recognize or identify with the feelings and needs of others** 7-NARCI 0 1 2 3

How do you feel when others start telling you about their
problems?

* Is it hard to put yourself in someone else's shoes and
understand what they're going through?
   (IF YES): Has this caused any problems for you?

Do other people say that you are not very sympathetic to their
problems?

11. **Requires excessive admiration** 4-NARCI 0 1 2 3

Is the praise and admiration of others important to you?
   (IF YES): Do you often feel empty and hurt because you
                  don't get the praise and admiration you think you
                  deserve?

12. **Is preoccupied with being criticized or rejected in social situations** 4-AVOID 0 1 2 3

In social situations, how much do you worry about being
criticized or rejected by other people?
   (IF A LOT): Are you able to get your mind off it?

13. **Appears indifferent to the praise or criticism of others** 6-SZOID 0 1 2 3

* How do you react when someone criticizes you?
   (IF NO REACTION):
                  So you don't look or feel upset after you've been
                  criticized?

* How do you react when someone compliments you?

Do you think about it later and feel good about it?

0=not present, 1=subthreshold, 2=present, 3=strongly present

---

14. Considers relationships to be more intimate than they actually are   8-HISTR   0 1 2 3

Do you often feel a close bond to someone you have just met?
(IF YES): Does this happen a lot?

* Do you sometimes get hurt in relationships because you think
the relationship is more serious than the other person does?

Do you often feel a close personal relationship with bosses or
professionals you haven't known very long?
(IF YES): Example?

---

15. Goes to excessive lengths to obtain nurturance and support from others, to the   5-DEPEN   0 1 2 3
point of volunteering to do things that are unpleasant

Do you bend over backward to do things for others because
you hope they'll take care of you when you need it?
(IF YES): Do you ever volunteer to do unpleasant things for
them because you hope they'll take care of you?

■ **(SKIP TO SECTION E IF OPTIONAL DIAGNOSES ARE NOT BEING ASSESSED)**

---

16. Complains of being misunderstood and unappreciated by others   2-NEGTV   0 1 2 3

---

* Do you often complain to others that people don't appreciate
or understand you?
(IF YES): How do they respond?

---

17. Unreasonably criticizes and scorns authority   4-NEGTV   0 1 2 3

Everyone must deal with people in charge, such as doctors,
teachers, employers, etc. Have the ones you've dealt with
generally done a pretty good job?
(IF NO): Are you often critical of your superiors?
Examples?

Are you disgusted with most of the authority figures you have
to deal with?

> **Scoring Guidelines:**
> *0 = not present or limited to rare isolated examples*
> *1 = subthreshold — some evidence of the trait, but it is not sufficiently*
> *pervasive or severe to consider the criterion present*
> *2 = present — criterion is clearly present for most of the last 5 years (i.e.,*
> *present at least 50% of the time during the last 5 years)*
> *3 = strongly present — criterion is associated with subjective distress or*
> *some impairment in social or occupational functioning or*
> *intimate relationships*

E. EMOTIONS

Now I would like to ask you some questions about your emotions.

---

1. Shows self-dramatization, theatricality, and exaggerated expression of emotion   6-HISTR   0 1 2 3

---

* Some people show their emotions easily. They cry at weddings,
embrace people, show their fear and their joy. Would you say
you're more or less likely than most people to show your
emotions?
   (IF MORE):   Has this ever caused you problems or
                    embarrassment?

Has anyone ever said anything about how you show your
emotions?
   (IF YES): What did they say?
                  Do you agree?

▋ **(RATING NOTE: ALSO CONSIDER EMOTIONAL EXPRESSIVENESS DURING INTERVIEW)**

---

2. Displays rapidly shifting and shallow expression of emotions   3-HISTR   0 1 2 3

---

* Do your emotions and feelings change quickly?
   (IF YES): Do other people notice?
                  Have you always been like that?

Has anyone ever commented that your emotions do not seem
real or sincere?
   (IF YES): Tell me about that.

---

3. Feels uncomfortable or helpless when alone because of exaggerated fears of   6-DEPEN   0 1 2 3
being unable to care for himself or herself

How do you usually feel when you're alone?
   (IF UNCOMFORTABLE):
                  What bothers you about being alone?
                  Are you often afraid that you won't be able to take
                  care of yourself?
                     (IF YES): In what way?

4. **Affective instability due to a marked reactivity of mood (e.g., intense episodic dysphoria, irritability, or anxiety usually lasting a few hours and only rarely more than a few days)**　　6-BORDL　　0　1　2　3

Do you often have days when your mood is constantly
changing — days when you shift back and forth from feeling
your usual self, to feeling angry or depressed or anxious?
　　(IF YES): Are the mood swings mild or are they very strong?
　　　　　　　How often does this happen in a typical week?
　　　　　　　How long do the moods last?

Has anyone ever told you that you're irritable or that your
moods seem to change a great deal?
　　(IF YES): Tell me about it.

5. **Chronic feelings of emptiness**　　7-BORDL　　0　1　2　3

Do you feel empty much of the time?
　　(IF YES): What percent of the time do you feel that way?

■ (SKIP TO SECTION F IF OPTIONAL DIAGNOSES ARE NOT BEING ASSESSED)

6. **Usual mood is dominated by dejection, gloominess, cheerlessness, joylessness, unhappiness**　　1-DEPRS　　0　1　2　3

* How would you describe your usual mood?
　　(IF UNCLEAR): Is it usually easy for you to laugh or smile?

Do you often feel gloomy or unhappy?
　　(IF DYSPHORIC):
　　　　　　　When did you start feeling this way?
　　　　　　　Have the times you have felt this way been limited
　　　　　　　to distinct periods of depression that are different
　　　　　　　from your usual self?

7. **Is prone to feeling guilty or remorseful**　　7-DEPRS　　0　1　2　3

* Are you quick to feel guilty or responsible whenever anything
goes wrong?
　　(IF YES): Do you feel this way even if other people don't
　　　　　　　blame you?

Do other people say you're too quick to apologize for anything
that goes wrong, even when it's not your fault?

Do you think you do this?

8. Is critical, blaming, and derogatory toward self	3-DEPRS	0 1 2 3

Would others say that you are too quick to blame yourself for anything that goes wrong?

Have you always been one to put yourself down and criticize yourself?

■ (RATING NOTE: USE RESPONSES TO ITEM #7 ON PREVIOUS PAGE TO RATE)

9. Following positive personal events (e.g., new achievement), responds with depression, guilt, or a behavior that produces pain (e.g., an accident)	3-SLFDF	0 1 2 3

When something good happens, do you often find yourself somehow feeling bad about it?
   (IF YES): What seems to make you feel bad?

When things are going well, do you often feel like you don't deserve it?
   (IF YES): Does this keep you from feeling good about it?

When something good happens to you, do you usually expect something bad to follow?

10. Alternates between hostile defiance and contrition	7-NEGTV	0 1 2 3

* Do you often tell somebody you won't do something, but then you end up feeling guilty and doing it anyway?

When you get up the nerve to tell someone off, do you often feel very guilty and take it all back afterward?

0=not present, 1=subthreshold, 2=present, 3=strongly present

> **Scoring Guidelines:**
> *0=not present or limited to rare isolated examples*
> *1=subthreshold — some evidence of the trait, but it is not sufficiently*
>   *pervasive or severe to consider the criterion present*
> *2=present — criterion is clearly present for most of the last 5 years (i.e.,*
>   *present at least 50% of the time during the last 5 years)*
> *3=strongly present — criterion is associated with subjective distress or*
>   *some impairment in social or occupational functioning or*
>   *intimate relationships*

F. OBSERVATIONAL CRITERIA

▮ ******* HALF-WAY POINT IN INTERVIEW ********

▮ NOTE: IN ORDER TO AVOID SUBJECT/INTERVIEWER FATIGUE, YOU MAY WISH TO
TAKE A BREAK HERE AND RATE THE ITEMS IN THIS SECTION, WHICH ARE BASED ON
YOUR OBSERVATIONS OF THE PATIENT RATHER THAN QUESTIONS YOU DIRECTLY
ASK THE PATIENT.

▮ THE QUESTIONS PRECEDED WITH AN ASTERISK (*) SHOULD BE ASKED OF THE
INFORMANT.

---

1. **Behavior or appearance that is odd, eccentric, or peculiar**   7-STYPL   0 1 2 3

* Is there anything odd or peculiar about the way (s)he looks?
     (IF YES): Describe.

* Does (s)he dress in an odd or peculiar way that is not
  explained by current fashion trends?
     (IF YES): Do you think (s)he dresses this way to attract
               attention or to fit in with friends?

     ▮ RATING NOTE: DO NOT RATE BEHAVIOR OR DRESS THAT IS INTENTIONALLY CHOSEN
     IN ORDER TO DRAW ATTENTION OR FIT IN, AS MAY OCCUR IN HISTRIONIC
     PERSONALITY DISORDER

* Does (s)he do odd or peculiar things?
     (IF YES): Describe.

* Does (s)he often talk to himself/herself?

---

2. **Odd thinking and speech (e.g., vague, circumstantial, metaphorical,**   4-STYPL   0 1 2 3
   overelaborate, or stereotyped)

---

* Does (s)he seem to talk in an odd or unusual way?
     (IF YES): How so?

* When (s)he talks about something, do you find it hard to
  follow what (s)he is saying?

3. Shows emotional coldness, detachment, or flattened affectivity	7-SZOID	0 1 2 3

* Does (s)he fail to show much facial or voice expression even when discussing material usually associated with some emotion?

* Is (s)he slow to look you in the eye when talking?

* Does (s)he usually smile or nod back at you during conversation?

* Does it seem like (s)he never expresses any emotion?

4. Inappropriate or constricted affect	6-STYPL	0 1 2 3

* Does it often seem like the emotion (s)he is showing does not fit with what (s)he is saying?

* Does (s)he often laugh or smile for no good reason?

■ (RATING NOTE: RATE CONSTRICTED AFFECT USING QUESTIONS FROM #3)

5. Has a style of speech that is excessively impressionistic and lacking in detail	5-HISTR	0 1 2 3

* Does (s)he give concrete examples with appropriate detail, especially when (s)he expresses a strong opinion?

0=not present, 1=subthreshold, 2=present, 3=strongly present

> **Scoring Guidelines:**
> *0=not present or limited to rare isolated examples*
> *1=subthreshold — some evidence of the trait, but it is not sufficiently pervasive or severe to consider the criterion present*
> *2=present — criterion is clearly present for most of the last 5 years (i.e., present at least 50% of the time during the last 5 years)*
> *3=strongly present — criterion is associated with subjective distress or some impairment in social or occupational functioning or intimate relationships*

G. SELF-PERCEPTION

The questions in this section ask about the way you think about yourself, and how you think others might describe you. Again, I am interested in the way you are when you are your usual self, not when you are experiencing an illness or are hospitalized.

---

1. **Identity disturbance: markedly and persistently unstable self-image or sense of self**   3-BORDL   0 1 2 3

Does the way you think about yourself change so often, that you don't know who you are anymore?
   (IF YES): Tell me what this is like.

Do you ever feel like you're someone else, or that you're evil, or maybe that you don't even exist?
   (IF YES): Tell me about that.

Some people think a lot about their sexual orientation, for instance, trying to decide whether or not they might be gay (or lesbian). Do you often worry about this?

---

2. **Has a sense of entitlement, i.e, unreasonable expectations of especially favorable treatment or automatic compliance with his or her expectations**   5-NARCI   0 1 2 3

Some people have earned the right to special treatment because of who they are or what they've done. Do you feel this way about yourself?
   (IF YES): Tell me about that.

Do you often get angry or irritated because you don't get the treatment you think you deserve?
   (IF YES): Examples?

* Do you have a reputation for expecting others to do whatever you say without questioning it?

3. Has a grandiose sense of self-importance (e.g., exaggerates achievements and talents, expects to be recognized as superior without commensurate achievements) 1-NARCI 0 1 2 3

Would you describe yourself as someone who has or will accomplish great things--accomplishments that will set you apart from your equals?
(IF YES): Tell me about them.

* Have people said you have too high an opinion of yourself?
(IF YES): Why do you think they said that?

4. Is preoccupied with fantasies of unlimited success, power, brilliance, beauty, or ideal love 2-NARCI 0 1 2 3

When people imagine what their life would be like if they could have anything they want, they may think of things like power, success, beauty, the perfect relationship, or other things. What do you daydream about?

If you were to add it all up, how much time do would you spend thinking about these things in a typical day?
#HOURS:_____.

Does daydreaming make it hard to concentrate on your work or get things done?

5. Is overconscientious, scrupulous, and inflexible about matters of morality, ethics, or values (not accounted for by cultural or religious identification) 4-OBCMP 0 1 2 3

* Are you more strict about moral and ethical values than most people you know?

Have other people complained that you're too strict about moral issues?
(IF YES): What did they complain about?

How often do you worry that you've done something immoral or unethical?

6. Shows rigidity and stubbornness 8-OBCMP 0 1 2 3

Would other people describe you as being stubborn or set in your ways?
(IF YES): What makes them say that?
Do you agree?

0=not present, 1=subthreshold, 2=present, 3=strongly present

---

7. **Is unable to discard worn-out or worthless objects even when they have no sentimental value**   5-OBCMP   0 1 2 3

Some people find it impossible to throw anything away, even
when it's old and worn out. Does this sound like you?
> **(IF YES):** What kinds of things do you keep?
> Why do you keep them?

Do others complain or tease you about the things you save?

---

8. **Is often envious of others or believes that others are envious of him or her**   8-NARCI   0 1 2 3

Are there people you really envy or are jealous of?
> **(IF YES):** What do you envy about them?
> How often do you think about this?
> Does thinking about this bother you a lot or keep
> you from getting things done?

Are people often jealous or envious of you?
> **(IF YES):** Why do you think they're jealous?

■ **(SKIP TO SECTION H IF OPTIONAL DIAGNOSES ARE NOT BEING ASSESSED)**

---

9. **Expresses envy and resentment toward those apparently more fortunate**   5-NEGTV   0 1 2 3

Do you often talk to others about how unfair it is that some
people are better off than you are?

■ **(RATING NOTE: USE RESPONSES TO ITEM #8 ABOVE TO RATE)**

---

10. **Engages in excessive self-sacrifice that is unsolicited by the intended recipients of the sacrifice**   8-SLFDF   0 1 2 3

---

*   How do you feel about doing favors for other people?

Do you feel like you do more for other people than they do for
you in return?
> **(IF YES):** Do you often go out of your way to help others
> even when they haven't asked for your help?

Do you sacrifice your own needs for the sake of others?
> **(IF YES):** Tell me about it.
> Has this been appreciated by others?
> Do they ask for these things?

11. Incites angry or rejecting responses from others and then feels hurt, defeated, or humiliated (e.g., makes fun of spouse in public, provoking an angry retort, then feels devastated)   4-SLFDF   0 1 2 3

Do you often do things that you know will make people angry
or cause them to reject you?
  (IF YES): What kinds of things do you do?
         How do you feel when they get angry or reject you?

12. Is negativistic, critical, and judgmental toward others   5-DEPRS   0 1 2 3

* Are you quick to criticize others?

Do you tend to notice people's faults more than their good
points?

When looking at things that most people admire, are you quick
to notice and point out the flaws?
  (IF YES): Example?

▌**(RATING NOTE: DO NOT RATE SELF-CRITICISM)**

13. Self-concept centers around beliefs of inadequacy, worthlessness, and low self-esteem   2-DEPRS   0 1 2 3

How would you describe your usual level of self-esteem?

When you compare yourself to other people, do you usually
feel like you're as good as others, or do you feel like they are
better than you?

14. Is pessimistic   6-DEPRS   0 1 2 3

* Are you usually an optimist or a pessimist?

Do you tend to expect the worst to happen?

15. Is sullen and argumentative   3-NEGTV   0 1 2 3

Does it often seem like every discussion turns into an
argument?

Do other people complain that they cannot have a discussion
with you without getting into an argument?

* On a scale of 1 to 10, where 1 is "usually grouchy," and 10 is
"usually cheerful," how do you think others would describe
you?

0=not present, 1=subthreshold, 2=present, 3=strongly present

16. Is brooding and given to worry   4-DEPRS   0 1 2 3

Are you the kind of person who always finds something to
worry about?

Do people tell you that you worry too much?

17. Voices exaggerated and persistent complaints of personal misfortune   6-NEGTV   0 1 2 3

Do you think you've had worse luck in life than most people?

* When you've had bad luck, are you quick to let others know, or
do you suffer in silence?

Do people ever complain that all you do is talk about your
problems?

Do others accuse you of exaggerating your problems?

▌ **(RATING NOTE: NOTICE WHETHER SUBJECT EXAGGERATES PROBLEMS IN OTHER
PARTS OF THE INTERVIEW)**

Scoring Guidelines:
0=not present or limited to rare isolated examples
1=subthreshold — some evidence of the trait, but it is not sufficiently
pervasive or severe to consider the criterion present
2=present — criterion is clearly present for most of the last 5 years (i.e.,
present at least 50% of the time during the last 5 years)
3=strongly present — criterion is associated with subjective distress or
some impairment in social or occupational functioning or
intimate relationships

H. PERCEPTION OF OTHERS

The questions in this section ask about experiences you may have had with other people. Remember that I'm interested in knowing how you feel about these situations when you are your usual self, not during an episode of illness or hospitalization.

---

1. Suspects, without sufficient basis, that others are exploiting, harming, or deceiving him or her
        1-PARND   0 1 2 3

Have you had experiences where people who pretended to be
your friends took advantage of you?
    (IF YES): What happened?
              How often has this happened?

Are you good at spotting someone who is trying to deceive or
con you?
    (IF YES): Examples?

---

2. Is preoccupied with unjustified doubts about the loyalty or trustworthiness of friends or associates
        2-PARND   0 1 2 3

---

* Are you concerned that certain friends or co-workers are not
really loyal or trustworthy?
    (IF YES): How much time do you spend thinking about this?
              What has caused your concern?

---

3. Perceives attacks on his or her character or reputation that are not apparent to others and is quick to react angrily or to counterattack
        6-PARND   0 1 2 3

Do you find that people often make indirect comments to
attack you or put you down, rather than tell you directly?
    (IF YES): How do you react?
              Do you get angry?
              Do you try to get back at the person?

4. **Reads hidden demeaning or threatening meanings into benign remarks or events**

                  4-PARND   0 1 2 3

Do people frequently seem to do things just to annoy you?
(**IF YES**): Examples?

Do you usually take what people tell you at face value, or do you frequently try to figure out what they really mean?
(**IF FIGURES OUT**):
        Do their comments often turn out to be hidden threats or put-downs?
                (**IF YES**): Explain?

* Do other people say that you read too much into situations and take offense at things that were not meant to be critical?
(**IF YES**): Example?

5. **Ideas of reference (excluding delusions of reference)**

                  1-STYPL   0 1 2 3

Have you ever found that people around you seem to be talking in general, but then you realize their comments are really meant for you?
(**IF YES**): How do you know they're talking about you?

Have you felt like someone in charge changed the rules specifically because of you, but they wouldn't admit it?

* Do you sometimes feel like strangers on the street are looking at you or talking about you?
(**IF YES**): Why do you think they notice you in particular?

6. **Is suggestible, i.e., easily influenced by others or circumstances**

                  7-HISTR   0 1 2 3

* Some people are so strongly influenced by others that they are easily swayed by their opinions. Do your opinions change easily depending on who you are with?
(**IF YES**): How often does this happen?

If someone says they have a problem such as a headache or upset stomach, or feels some strong emotion, do you suddenly feel the same way?
(**IF YES**): Example?

---

7. **Odd beliefs or magical thinking that influences behavior and is inconsistent with subcultural norms (e.g., superstitiousness, belief in clairvoyance, telepathy, or "sixth sense"; in children and adolescents, bizarre fantasies or preoccupations)** 2-STYPL 0 1 2 3

A number of people talk about telepathy or ESP and feel like they can sense what's in someone's mind or predict the future. Have you had any experiences like this?
(IF YES): Examples?
Have your friends and family also had experiences like this?
Are these experiences very important to your life?
(IF YES): How?

Are you a superstitious person?
(IF YES): In what way?
How does this influence your decisions or what you do?
Do your friends and family share these superstitions?

Some people believe they can influence things like the weather or ball games just by thinking about them. Do you believe that you can make things happen just by thinking about them?
(IF YES): Tell me about it.

* Do you believe in hexes, curses, omens, voodoo, or other things like this?
(IF YES): Have any of these things influenced your decisions or behavior?
Do your friends and family share these beliefs?

---

8. **Unusual perceptual experiences, including bodily illusions** 3-STYPL 0 1 2 3

Have you ever sensed there was some unusual force or presence in the room?
(IF YES): Can you describe what this was like?
What do you think caused this?
How often has this happened?

Have you ever felt like you or the world around you looked or seemed different than it usually does?
(IF YES): What was this like?
Were you using any drugs or alcohol at the time?

Do your eyes ever play tricks on you--for instance, your or someone else's face or body looks different?
(IF YES): Can you tell me about this?

---

9. **Suspiciousness or paranoid ideation** 5-STYPL 0 1 2 3

(RATE ITEM POSITIVE IF ANY 2 OF THE CRITERIA FOR PARANOID PERSONALITY DISORDER ARE PRESENT ON THE SCORESHEET, EXCLUDING CRITERION #5)

0=not present, 1=subthreshold, 2=present, 3=strongly present

Scoring Guidelines:
0=not present or limited to rare isolated examples
*1=subthreshold — some evidence of the trait, but it is not sufficiently
        pervasive or severe to consider the criterion present*
*2=present — criterion is clearly present for most of the last 5 years (i.e.,
        present at least 50% of the time during the last 5 years)*
*3=strongly present — criterion is associated with subjective distress or
        some impairment in social or occupational functioning or
        intimate relationships*

I. STRESS AND ANGER

This section asks about the way you usually express anger or react to stressful situations. Remember that I am interested in how you react when you are your usual self.

---

1. **Inappropriate, intense anger or difficulty controlling anger (e.g., frequent displays of temper, constant anger, recurrent physical fights)**   8-BORDL   0 1 2 3

---

* How often do you lose your temper?

   What kinds of things get you really angry?

* Tell me what you're like when you are very angry.

   How long do you usually stay angry?

   Do you throw or break things?

   Have you hit anyone while you were angry?

   Do you ever get into physical fights?

   When you're angry, do you ever give someone the silent treatment?
   (IF YES): How long can you keep it up?
            Is that a common reaction for you?

   Are there times when you feel very angry, but don't show it?
   (IF YES): How much of the time do you feel angry?

---

2. **Shows arrogant, haughty behaviors or attitudes**   9-NARCI   0 1 2 3

Have other people told you that you have an attitude problem?
   (IF YES): What did they mean?

▮ **(RATING NOTE: ALSO CONSIDER BEHAVIOR DURING INTERVIEW)**

---

3. Persistently bears grudges, i.e., is unforgiving of insults, injuries, or slights   5-PARND   0 1 2 3

How long would you stay angry at someone who does
something to hurt or insult you, like forgetting your birthday?

Do you tend to hold grudges?
Are there any people you've never forgiven?
   (IF YES TO EITHER):
           Can you tell me about it?

---

4. Transient, stress-related paranoid ideation or severe dissociative symptoms   9-BORDL   0 1 2 3

When some people are under stress, they may have
experiences that are very hard to explain to other people. For
example, when you're under stress, have you ever felt like
things around you were somehow strange, or changed in size
or shape?
   (IF YES): Describe what that is like.

When you've been under stress, have you ever felt like your
body or a part of it was somehow changed or not real?

Have you ever felt like you were watching yourself from
outside your body?
   (IF YES): Describe what that was like.

Do you ever have brief blackouts and forget what has
happened?

When you're feeling stressed, do you ever get paranoid or
suspicious of people you usually trust?
   (IF NO):   What about being afraid that someone is spying on
                  you or planning to hurt you?

■ **(IF ANY OF ABOVE ARE POSITIVE, ASK):**

You've said that you've experienced [*list dissociative or
paranoid experiences*]: Were you using drugs or alcohol when
this happened?
   (IF YES): Does this happen only when you're using drugs or
                  alcohol?
   (IF OCCURS WHEN NOT USING DRUGS OR ALCOHOL):
           How long do these experiences last?
           Does this happen when you are not under stress?

5.   Recurrent suicidal behavior, gestures, or threats, or self-mutilating behavior   5-BORDL   0   1   2   3

Have you ever been so upset that you told someone you
wanted to hurt or kill yourself?
    (IF YES): Tell me about it.
             How often have you done this?

*   Have you ever made a suicide attempt, even one that didn't
cause serious injury?
    (IF YES): What did you do?
             How many attempts have you made?

Have you ever been so upset or tense that you deliberately
hurt yourself by cutting your skin, putting your hand through a
glass window, burning yourself, or anything else like that?
    (IF YES): What have you done?
             How often?

Scoring Guidelines:
0=not present or limited to rare isolated examples
1=subthreshold — some evidence of the trait, but it is not sufficiently pervasive or severe to consider the criterion present
2=present — criterion is clearly present for most of the last 5 years (i.e., present at least 50% of the time during the last 5 years)
3=strongly present — criterion is associated with subjective distress or some impairment in social or occupational functioning or intimate relationships

J. SOCIAL CONFORMITY

1. **Impulsivity in at least two areas that are potentially self-damaging (e.g., spending, sex, substance abuse, reckless driving, binge eating) [Note: Do not include suicidal or self-mutilating behavior covered in Criterion 5]**   4-BORDL   0 1 2 3

I am going to read you a list of behaviors that sometimes cause problems for people. In the past 5 years, how many times have you:

*   1. ___gambled more money than you could afford to lose?
*   2. ___bought unnecessary things you could not afford?
*   3. ___had one-night stands or brief sexual affairs?
*   4. ___been intoxicated on alcohol?
*   5. ___been stoned or high on other drugs?
*   6. ___shoplifted or took something that didn't belong to you?
*   7. ___been in an auto accident, received a speeding ticket, or been charged with reckless driving?
*   8. ___driven while intoxicated or high?
*   9. ___gone on eating binges where you ate so much food that you had stomach pain or you had to throw up?
*   10. ___done anything else impulsive where you could have gotten hurt?

▐ **(SKIP THE REMAINDER OF THIS SECTION IF ANTISOCIAL PERSONALITY DISORDER IS BEING SCREENED BY SOME OTHER INSTRUMENT)**

2. **Irritability and aggressiveness, as indicated by repeated physical fights or assaults**   4-ANTSO   0 1 2 3

▐ **(RATING NOTE: USE RESPONSES TO ITEM #1 IN SECTION I, PAGE 27, TO RATE)**

3. **Failure to conform to social norms with respect to lawful behaviors as indicated by repeatedly performing acts that are grounds for arrest**   1-ANTSO   0 1 2 3

I am not interested in knowing any specific details, but I need to ask how many times you might have done any of the following...
>   **(IF AGE <20)**   ...between age 15 and your current age:
>   **(IF AGE >20)**   ...in the last 5 years:

>   ____bought or sold stolen property
>   ____embezzled other people's money
>   ____ran numbers
>   ____sold drugs
>   ____shoplifted or stolen things
>   ____had sex for money
>   ____done other things that could have gotten you arrested

*Have you ever been arrested?
>   **(IF YES)**: How many times?
>   What were the circumstances?

4. **Consistent irresponsibility, as indicated by repeated failure to sustain consistent work behavior or honor financial obligations**   6-ANTSO   0 1 2 3

>   Have you been unable to pay for necessities such as food, rent, or the electric bill because you spent so much money on things you could have done without?

*   Have you sometimes not paid bills or other financial obligations?
>   **(IF YES)**: What were the circumstances?

>   Have you ever failed to make court-ordered payments such as child support, alimony, or a lawsuit settlement?
>   **(IF YES)**: Tell me about it.

>   When you're working, have you ever gotten into trouble for not arriving on time, missing too many days, not doing your work, or not following the rules?
>   **(IF YES)**: Tell me about that.

5. **Deceitfulness, as indicated by repeated lying, use of aliases, or conning others for personal profit or pleasure**   2-ANTSO   0 1 2 3

*   Is it easy for you to lie if it serves your purpose?

>   Have you ever used a false name or developed a scheme to con people into giving you what you want?

31

6. Impulsivity or failure to plan ahead   3-ANTSO   0 1 2 3

How often have you just walked off a job or quit without a
specific plan?
(IF PRESENT): Tell me about it.

How often have you moved around from place to place without
any idea of how long you would stay or where you would go
next?
(IF PRESENT): Tell me about it.

* Do you often get into trouble because you don't plan ahead?
(IF YES): Examples?

■ **(REFER TO QUESTION #1 IN THIS SECTION FOR ADDITIONAL RELATED BEHAVIORS)**

---

7. Reckless disregard for safety of self or others   5-ANTSO   0 1 2 3

Are you known as someone who risks life and limb in
recreational activities?
(IF YES): How did you get this reputation?

Did you ever get into trouble at work for doing things that
could be dangerous to you or others?
(IF YES): What happened?

■ **(REFER TO QUESTION #1 IN THIS SECTION FOR ADDITIONAL RELATED BEHAVIORS)**

---

8. Lack of remorse, as indicated by being indifferent to or rationalizing having hurt,   7-ANTSO   0 1 2 3
mistreated, or stolen from another

■ **(SKIP THIS QUESTION IF NO ANTISOCIAL BEHAVIORS WERE ELICITED)**

You mentioned that you have [*summarize antisocial behaviors,
especially violating rights of others*]. How do you feel about that?
(IF NO REMORSE):
        Do you ever feel sorry or guilty?
        Do you often feel that your actions were justified
        by the situation?
            (IF YES): Explain?

0=not present, 1=subthreshold, 2=present, 3=strongly present

9. Evidence of Conduct Disorder with onset before age 15 years

C-ANTSO   0 1 2 3

▍**(THIS SECTION CAN BE SKIPPED IF NO SUBSTANTIAL ADULT ANTISOCIAL CRITERIA WERE PRESENT)**

In order to understand how your current situation relates to certain childhood behaviors, I need to ask how many times you did the following before you were 15 years old:

Before the age of 15, how many times did you:

1. ___stay out much later than your parents said you should?
2. ___skip school?
3. ___run away from home overnight?
     (IF ONLY ONCE): Did you return home to live after running away?
4. ___threaten or pick on other kids?
5. ___start physical fights?
6. ___use a knife, gun, bat, or anything else that could hurt someone?
7. ___purposely hurt other people when you were not in a fight?
8. ___purposely hurt an animal?
9. ___force someone to have sex with you?
10. ___purposely damage someone's property?
11. ___intentionally start a fire that caused serious damage?
12. ___get in trouble for lying or breaking promises?
13. ___steal from stores, your parents, or other people?
14. ___rob or threaten anyone if they didn't give you something you wanted?
15. ___break into someone else's home, building, or car?

▍**(CRITERION C FOR ANTISOCIAL PERSONALITY DISORDER IS MET IF 3 OR MORE OF THE ABOVE WERE CLEARLY PRESENT)**

CONSENT TO CONTACT A RELATIVE, FRIEND, OR OTHER INDIVIDUAL

By signing this form you are giving us permission to talk to someone who knows you well, in order to better understand your personality. If you give us permission to contact someone, we will not discuss your answers with them. We will ask them a shorter series of questions, similar to the questions that we ask you.

I _____ give my permission for
      (print name of person evaluated)

_____ or his/her assistants
     (print name of clinician)

to contact the following person(s) in order to ask questions about what I am usually like and what kinds of situations may cause problems for me. I understand that you will not discuss my answers with them.

	NAME	RELATIONSHIP	PHONE (Best Time to Call)
1.	_____	_____	_____
2.	_____	_____	_____
3.	_____	_____	_____

This permission automatically expires in 1 year.

_____   _____
Signature   Date

_____
Witness

SIDP-IV SCORESHEET

Name _____ # _____ Date ___/___/___

Age _____

Gender: M F

Marital: Married Widowed Separated Divorced Never married

Axis I _____

Interviewer: _____

General Diagnostic Criteria for a Personality Disorder (GCPD)

DSM-IV requires that the following be present in order to diagnose a personality disorder:

[ ] A. An enduring pattern of inner experience and behavior that deviates markedly from the expectations of the individual's culture. This pattern is manifested in two (or more) of the following areas:

( ) 1. cognition (i.e., ways of perceiving and interpreting self, other people, and events

( ) 2. affectivity (i.e., the range, intensity, lability, and appropriateness of emotional response)

( ) 3. interpersonal functioning

( ) 4. impulse control

[ ] B. The enduring pattern is inflexible and pervasive across a broad range of personal and social situations

[ ] C. The enduring pattern leads to clinically significant distress or impairment in social, occupational, or other important areas of functioning

[ ] D. The pattern is stable and of long duration and its onset can be traced back at least to adolescence or early adulthood**

[ ] E. The enduring pattern is not better accounted for as a manifestation or consequence of another mental disorder (e.g., the personality disorders exclude a personality disorder if personality problems are explained by schizophrenia, a mood disorder with psychotic features, or another psychotic disorder)

[ ] F. The enduring pattern is not due to the direct physiological effects of a substance (e.g., a drug of abuse, a medication) or a general medical condition (e.g., head trauma)

** Criterion D will generally be operationalized using the "5-year rule" (see SIDP instructions at beginning of booklet). This means that a trait will be considered "stable and of long duration" if it has been present for most of the last 5 years. Cases in which personality functioning during the last 5 years represents a deterioration from earlier functioning will usually be excluded from personality diagnosis by Criterion E, since the onset of a clearly defined Axis I disorder will usually be the cause.

301.82 Avoidant (AVOID)

[ ] A. 4 or more of following plus GCPD:

( ) 1. avoids occupational activities that involve significant interpersonal contact, because of fears of criticism, disapproval, or rejection (p. 4)

( ) 2. is unwilling to get involved with people unless certain of being liked (p. 11)

( ) 3. shows restraint within intimate relationships because of the fear of being shamed or ridiculed (p. 7)

( ) 4. is preoccupied with being criticized or rejected in social situations (p. 12)

( ) 5. is inhibited in new interpersonal situations because of feelings of inadequacy (p. 11)

( ) 6. views self as socially inept, personally unappealing, or inferior to others (p. 10)

( ) 7. is unusually reluctant to take personal risks or to engage in any new activities because they may prove embarrassing (p. 1)

301.6 Dependent (DEPEN)

[ ] A. 5 or more of following plus GCPD:

( ) 1. has difficulty making everyday decisions without an excessive amount of advice and reassurance from others (p. 2)

( ) 2. needs others to assume responsibility for most major areas of his or her life (p. 2)

( ) 3. has difficulty expressing disagreement with others because of fear of loss of support or approval (p. 7)

( ) 4. has difficulty initiating projects or doing things on his or her own (because of a lack of self-confidence in judgment or abilities rather than a lack of motivation or energy) (p. 2)

( ) 5. goes to excessive lengths to obtain nurturance and support from others, to the point of volunteering to do things that are unpleasant (p. 13)

( ) 6. feels uncomfortable or helpless when alone because of exaggerated fears of being unable to care for himself or herself (p. 14)

( ) 7. urgently seeks another relationship as a source of care and support when a close relationship ends (p. 8)

( ) 8. is unrealistically preoccupied with fears of being left to take care of himself or herself (p. 8)

301.4 Obsessive-Compulsive (OBCMP)

[ ] A. 4 or more of following plus GCPD:

( ) 1. is preoccupied with details, rules, lists, order, organization, or schedules to the extent that the major point of the activity is lost (p. 5)

( ) 2. shows perfectionism that interferes with task completion (p. 5)

( ) 3. is excessively devoted to work and productivity to the exclusion of leisure activities and friendships (p. 4)

( ) 4. is overconscientious, scrupulous, and inflexible about matters of morality, ethics, or values (not accounted for by cultural or religious identification) (p. 20)

( ) 5. is unable to discard worn-out or worthless objects even when they have no sentimental value (p. 21)

( ) 6. is reluctant to delegate tasks or to work with others unless they submit to exactly his or her way of doing things (p. 5)

( ) 7. adopts a miserly spending style toward both self and others; money is viewed as something to be hoarded for future catastrophes (p. 2)

( ) 8. shows rigidity and stubbornness (p. 20)

301.9S Self-Defeating (SLFDF) — optional

[ ] A. 5 or more of following plus GCPD:

( ) 1. chooses people and situations that lead to disappointment, failure, or mistreatment even when better options are clearly available (p. 9)

( ) 2. rejects or renders ineffective the attempts of others to help him or her (p. 6)

( ) 3. following positive personal events, responds with depression, guilt, or behavior producing pain (p. 16)

( ) 4. incites angry or rejecting responses from others and then feels hurt, defeated, or humiliated (p. 22)

( ) 5. rejects opportunities for pleasure, or is reluctant to acknowledge enjoying himself or herself (despite having adequate social skills and the capacity for pleasure) (p. 3)

( ) 6. fails to accomplish tasks crucial to his or her personal objectives despite demonstrated ability to do so, e.g., helps fellow students write papers, but is unable to write his/her own (p. 6)

( ) 7. is uninterested in or rejects people who consistently treat him or her well (p. 9)

( ) 8. engages in excessive self-sacrifice that is unsolicited by the intended recipients of the sacrifice (p. 21)

301.9D Depressive (DEPRS) — optional

[ ] A. 5 or more of following plus GCPD:

( ) 1. usual mood is dominated by dejection, gloominess, cheerlessness, joylessness, unhappiness (p. 15)

( ) 2. self-concept centers around beliefs of inadequacy, worthlessness, and low self-esteem (p. 22)

( ) 3. is critical, blaming, and derogatory toward self (p. 16)

( ) 4. is brooding and given to worry (p. 23)

( ) 5. is negativistic, critical, and judgmental (p. 22)

( ) 6. is pessimistic (p. 22)

( ) 7. is prone to feeling guilty or remorseful (p. 15)

301.9N Negativistic (NEGTV) — optional

[ ] A. 4 or more of following plus GCPD:

( ) 1. passively resists fulfilling routine social and occupational tasks (p. 6)

( ) 2. complains of being misunderstood and unappreciated by others (p. 13)

( ) 3. is sullen and argumentative (p. 22)

( ) 4. unreasonably criticizes and scorns authority (p. 13)

( ) 5. expresses envy and resentment toward those apparently more fortunate (p. 21)

( ) 6. voices exaggerated and persistent complaints of personal misfortune (p. 23)

( ) 7. alternates between hostile defiance and contrition (p. 16)

301.9M Mixed (MIXED)

[ ] A. Patient meets criteria for GCPD

[ ] B. Patient comes within one criterion of meeting two or more personality disorders from the 10 nonoptional personality disorders

[ ] C. Does not meet full criteria for any other personality disorder

SEE NEXT PAGE FOR SUGGESTIONS ON COMPUTER CODING CONVENTIONS

Suggested Computer Coding Variable Names

In order to facilitate the exchange of data between different centers using the SIDP-IV, the following conventions are suggested for variable names when coding SIDP interview data:

Each of the criteria under a specific personality diagnosis will be designated by the 5-letter code for that disorder (see previous 2 pages) followed by the criterion number. For example, the seven criteria for paranoid personality disorder would be coded as PARND1, PARND2, PARND3...PARND7. The values for each of these variables would be 0 = not present, 1 = subthreshold, 2 = present, 3 = strongly present, and -9 = missing data.

The letter A will be added to each 5-digit code to create a variable that indicates the overall presence or absence of each disorder, for example, PARNDA = 1 indicates criteria are met for paranoid personality disorder. If insufficient criteria are met, then PARNDA = 0. Likewise BORDLA = 1 indicates that sufficient criteria were present to diagnose borderline personality disorder. A value of -9 can be used to indicate missing data, e.g., PARNDA = -9.

The letter N can be added to each 5-digit code to record the total number of criteria that were scored 2 or higher for that disorder. For example, ANTSON = 4 would indicate that 4 of the 7 antisocial criteria were scored as 2 or more. In order to record scores for each of the personality clusters, the following computer codes are suggested:

CLSTAN = PARNDN + SZOIDN + STYPLN
CLSTBN = ANTSON + BORDLN + HISTRN + NARCIN
CLSTCN = AVOIDN + DEPENN + OBCMPN
TOTCRN = CLSTAN + CLSTBN + CLSTCN

ANYPD = 1 if any of the first 10 (nonoptional) personality disorders are present.
OPTIN = 1 if any of the optional personality disorders are present. OPTIN = 0 if none of these disorders are met, and OPTIN = -9 if these data are missing or unavailable.

If desired, the GCPD criteria A through F may be coded as GCPDA, GCPDB...GCPDF with 1 = present and 0 = absent. Sub-criteria under GCPDA would be coded as GCPDA1...GCPDA4.

The following variable names are suggested for general demographic information (*information can be coded in space provided before each variable name for easy computer entry*):

___ AGE   subject's age at time of interview
___ SEX   1 = male, 2 = female
___ EDUC   number of years of education
___ STATUS   1 = not currently receiving inpatient or outpatient psychiatric treatment
                  2 = currently receiving outpatient mental health care or follow-up
                  3 = hospitalized as a psychiatric patient at the time of interview
                  4 = in a partial hospitalization program or other institutional living situation
___ MARITAL 1 = married, 2 = widowed, 3 = separated, 4 = divorced, 5 = never married

Previous attempts to combine SIDP data sets from different centers have been limited by a lack of consistent coding of Axis I disorders. The following brief list of Axis I variable names and codes is intended as a rudimentary means of summarizing Axis I data. The space in front of each variable name may be used to record the applicable code for a given subject to provide for future reference or computer data entry. The quality of this data will depend on the methods used to assess Axis I.

___ MJDEP — major depression
___ DYSTH — dysthymia
___ BIPL1 — bipolar type I
___ BIPL2 — bipolar type II

___ PANIC — panic disorder
___ GENAX — generalized anxiety disorder
___ SOCPH — social phobia
___ OCDX1 — obsessive-compulsive disorder (on Axis I)
___ PTSDD — posttraumatic stress disorder

___ ALCHL — alcohol abuse or dependence
___ SUBST — substance abuse other than alcohol

___ ANORX — anorexia nervosa
___ BULIM — bulimia nervosa

___ SCPHR — schizophrenia
___ SCZAF — schizoaffective disorder
___ DELUS — delusional disorder

___ SOMAT — somatization disorder
___ DISID — dissociative identity disorder
___ DISOC — other dissociative disorder

___ GENMD — a general medical condition (e.g., Down's syndrome, stroke, hyperthyroidism) is the direct cause of a psychiatric disturbance

Each of the above Axis I variables can be coded as follows:

0 = diagnosis absent in past and present

1 = subject met criteria for this Axis I disorder at the time of the SIDP-IV interview

2 = subject has met criteria for this Axis I disorder in the past but not at the time of this interview

5 = evidence exists for a probable or atypical form of this Axis I disorder

-9 = missing data

301.00 Paranoid (PARND)

[ ] A. 4 or more of following plus GCPD:

(   ) 1. suspects, without sufficient basis, that others are exploiting or deceiving him or her (p. 24)

(   ) 2. is preoccupied with unjustified doubts about the loyalty or trustworthiness of friends or associates (p. 24)

(   ) 3. is reluctant to confide in others because of unwarranted fear that the information will be used maliciously against him or her (p. 12)

(   ) 4. reads hidden demeaning or threatening meanings into benign remarks or events (p. 25)

(   ) 5. persistently bears grudges, i.e., unforgiving of insults, injuries, or slights (p. 28)

(   ) 6. perceives attacks on his or her character or reputation that are not apparent to others and is quick to react angrily or counterattack (p. 24)

(   ) 7. has recurrent suspicions, without justification, regarding fidelity of spouse or sexual partner (p. 9)

301.20 Schizoid (SZOID)

[ ] A. 4 or more of following plus GCPD:

(   ) 1. neither desires nor enjoys close relationships, including being part of a family (p. 7)

(   ) 2. almost always chooses solitary activities (p. 1)

(   ) 3. has little if any interest in having sexual experiences with another person (p. 9)

(   ) 4. takes pleasure in few, if any, activities (p. 1)

(   ) 5. lacks close friends or confidants other than first-degree relatives (p. 7)

(   ) 6. appears indifferent to praise or criticism (p. 12)

(   ) 7. shows emotional coldness, detachment, or flattened affectivity (p. 18)

301.22 Schizotypal (STYPL)

[ ] A. 5 or more of following plus GCPD:

(   ) 1. ideas of reference (p. 25)

(   ) 2. odd beliefs or magical thinking, influencing behavior and inconsistent with subcultural norms (p. 26)

(   ) 3. unusual perceptual experiences, including bodily illusions (p. 26)

(   ) 4. odd thinking and speech (p. 17)

(   ) 5. suspiciousness or paranoid ideation (p. 26)

(   ) 6. inappropriate or constricted affect (p. 18)

(   ) 7. behavior or appearance that is odd, eccentric, or peculiar (p. 17)

(   ) 8. lack of close friends or confidants other than first-degree relatives (p. 7)

(   ) 9. excessive social anxiety that does not diminish with familiarity and tends to be associated with paranoid fears rather than negative judgments about self (p. 11)

301.7 Antisocial (ANTSO)

[ ] A. 3 or more of following, B, C, plus GCPD:

(   ) 1. failure to conform to social norms with respect to lawful behaviors as indicated by repeatedly performing acts that are grounds for arrest (p. 31)

(   ) 2. deceitfulness, as indicated by repeated lying, use of aliases, or conning others for personal profit or pleasure (p. 31)

(   ) 3. impulsivity or failure to plan ahead (p. 32)

(   ) 4. irritability and aggressiveness, as indicated by repeated physical fights or assaults (p. 30)

(   ) 5. reckless disregard for safety of self or others (p. 32)

(   ) 6. consistent irresponsibility, as indicated by repeated failure to sustain consistent work behavior or honor financial obligations (p. 31)

(   ) 7. lack of remorse, as indicated by being indifferent to, or rationalizing having hurt, mistreated, or stolen from another (p. 32)

[ ] B. The individual is at least 18 years of age

[ ] C. There is evidence of Conduct Disorder with onset before age 15 (p. 33)

301.83 Borderline (BORDL)

[ ] A. 5 or more of following plus GCPD:

(   ) 1. frantic efforts to avoid real or imagined abandonment (p. 8)

(   ) 2. a pattern of unstable and intense interpersonal relationships characterized by alternating between extremes of idealization and devaluation (p. 8)

(   ) 3. identity disturbance: markedly and persistently unstable self-image or sense of self (p. 19)

(   ) 4. impulsivity in at least two areas that are potentially self-damaging (e.g., spending, sex, substance abuse, reckless driving, binge eating) (p. 30)

(   ) 5. recurrent suicidal behavior, gestures, or threats, or self-mutilating behavior (p. 29)

(   ) 6. affective instability/marked reactivity of mood (p. 15)

(   ) 7. chronic feelings of emptiness (p. 15)

(   ) 8. inappropriate, intense anger or difficulty controlling anger (p. 27)

(   ) 9. transient, stress-related paranoid ideation or severe dissociative symptoms (p. 28)

301.50 Histrionic (HISTR)

[ ] A. 5 or more of following plus GCPD:

(   ) 1. is uncomfortable in situations in which he or she is not the center of attention (p. 10)

(   ) 2. interaction with others is often characterized by inappropriate sexually seductive or provocative behavior (p. 10)

(   ) 3. displays rapidly shifting and shallow expression of emotion (p. 14)

(   ) 4. consistently uses physical appearance to draw attention to self (p. 11)

(   ) 5. style of speech that is excessively impressionistic and lacking in detail (p. 18)

(   ) 6. shows self-dramatization, theatricality, and exaggerated expression of emotion (p. 14)

(   ) 7. is suggestible, i.e., easily influenced by others or circumstances (p. 25)

(   ) 8. considers relationships to be more intimate than they actually are (p. 13)

301.81 Narcissistic (NARCI)

[ ] A. 5 or more of following plus GCPD:

(   ) 1. has a grandiose sense of self-importance (p. 20)

(   ) 2. is preoccupied with fantasies of unlimited success, power, brilliance, beauty, or ideal love (p. 20)

(   ) 3. believes he or she is "special" and unique and can only be understood by other special or high-status people (p. 11)

(   ) 4. requires excessive admiration (p. 12)

(   ) 5. has a sense of entitlement (p. 19)

(   ) 6. is interpersonally exploitative, i.e., takes advantage of others to achieve his or her own ends (p. 5)

(   ) 7. lacks empathy: unwilling to recognize or identify with the feelings and needs of others (p. 12)

(   ) 8. is often envious of others or believes that others are envious of him or her (p. 21)

(   ) 9. shows arrogant, haughty behaviors or attitudes (p. 27)

0=not present, 1=subthreshold, 2=present, 3=strongly present

"I have utilized the SIDP-IV as a diagnostic tool from its inception, and I have found it to be of exceptional value in diagnosing personality disorders. There are several improvements in this version, including the use of topical sections and questions that are formulated in such a way as to cover a wider range of experience instead of a narrow focus on symptoms."

Larry J. Siever, M.D.
Professor of Psychiatry
Director of Special Evaluation Program for Mood and
    Personality Disorders
Mt. Sinai School of Medicine and Bronx VA Medical Centers
Bronx, New York

"The SIDP-IV is the one structured interview that I have consistently recommended for research projects oriented to the analysis of personality disorders. Combined with a psychometrically sensitive self-report inventory, it can prove of value also as a tool for clinical assessment."

Theodore Millon, Ph.D., D.Sc.
Professor of Psychiatry, Harvard Medical School
Professor of Psychology, University of Miami
Miami, Florida

"The SIDP-IV is a very "user-friendly" semistructured interview for diagnosing DSM-IV personality disorders. It can readily be used in both research and clinical situations. The SIDP-IV provides the interviewer with the specific criterion being measured followed by appropriate nonbiased probes that can be elaborated upon by the interviewer. The scoring is easy and straightforward. The criteria are not clustered by diagnoses; rather, they are sorted into 10 functional categories that allow a coherence and a smoothness to the interview. The interview's probes and structure make excellent clinical sense while providing an operationalized method for more accurate diagnosis of these difficult and confusing disorders."

Kenneth R. Silk, M.D.
Associate Chair for Clinical and Administrative Affairs
Director, Personality Disorders Section
Adult Ambulatory Division
Department of Psychiatry
University of Michigan Medical Center
Ann Arbor, Michigan

ISBN 978-0-88048-937-9
90000

9 780880 489379

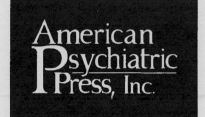

American
Psychiatric
Press, Inc.